Alkaline Diet

The Comprehensive And Concise Guide For Novices On
The Impact Of Food On The Acid-alkaline Balance Of The
Body, With The Objective Of Disease Reversal And
Weight Reduction

Desmond Slater

TABLE OF CONTENT

Introduction

This book contains proven steps and strategies on how to lose weight while making your body healthier. There is a multitude of food items consumed in contemporary society that have detrimental effects on individuals' health. Ill individuals ultimately allocate their diligently earned funds towards healthcare expenses. There is no longer a need for you to experience physical discomfort. This book presents a comprehensive approach to nutrition that will enable you to cultivate a nourishing diet, ultimately leading to a robust and invigorated physical well-being. There is hope. It is not necessary to meticulously track calorie intake or dedicate extensive hours at the gym in order to achieve weight loss. Through the adoption of this nutritious dietary regimen, you will inevitably ascertain that achieving weight loss and experiencing enhanced well-being can be accomplished sans any substantial feelings of hunger.

Thank you once again for downloading this book. I sincerely hope that you derive great pleasure from it.

This document aims to deliver precise and trustworthy information pertaining to the discussed subject matter and concern. The publication is marketed on the premise that the publisher is exempt from providing accounting, officially sanctioned, or any other type of expert services. In the event that guidance or counsel is deemed essential, it is advisable to engage the services of an experienced practitioner in the respective field, particularly if the matter pertains to legal or professional affairs.

- Derived from a Declaration of Principles that garnered equal acceptance and approval from both a Committee of the American Bar Association and a Committee of Publishers and Associations.

The information presented in this document is intended to be accurate and reliable. The recipient reader bears sole and complete responsibility for any negligence or misuse of the policies, procedures, or instructions outlined herein. The publisher shall not incur any legal liability or culpability, in any circumstance, for any restitution, harm, or financial detriment arising from the information contained herein, whether directly or indirectly.

The publisher does not hold the copyrights for the respective authors.

The information contained herein is provided exclusively for informational purposes, and is applicable universally. The information presented does not come with any contractual obligations or guarantees of any kind.

The trademarks utilized are non-consensual, and the publication of said trademarks lacks authorization or endorsement from the trademark proprietor. The trademarks and brands mentioned in this book are solely for illustrative purposes and belong to their respective owners. They are not affiliated with or endorsed by this document.

What does the Alkaline Diet entail?

A diet aimed at reducing acidity places an emphasis on consuming alkaline foods, such as fresh produce and specific types of whole grains, that are characterized by their low caloric density. Prominent examples of Alkaline Diet Foods exemplify a fine balance between foods that promote acidity and those that encourage alkalinity.

The human body comprises diverse organ systems that are adept at neutralizing and eliminating excessive acidity. However, there exists a threshold beyond which even a healthy body cannot effectively manage an excessive amount of acid.

The human body possesses the capability to maintain an acid-alkaline equilibrium provided that the organs are functioning optimally, a properly balanced alkaline diet is being consumed, and other factors that contribute to acid production, such as tobacco use, are avoided.

The antacid consumption regimen significantly diminishes this acid load, thereby helping to reduce the burden on the body's acid detoxification systems, such as the kidneys.

Presented below is an overview of Alkaline Foods, with special focus on High Alkaline Foods:

Examples of Alkalizing Vegetables: Beetroot, Brassica oleracea (including broccoli and cauliflower), Apium graveolens, Cucumis sativus, Brassica oleracea var. sabellica (kale), Lactuca sativa, Allium cepa, Pisum sativum, Capsicum annuum, Spinacia oleracea

Evidence of Alkalizing Fruits: Apple, Banana, Berries, Cantaloupe, Grapes, Melon, Lemon, Orange, Peach, Pear, Watermelon

Examples of Alkaline-Protein Sources: Almonds, Chestnuts, and Tofu

Spices that promote alkalinity: Cinnamon, curry, ginger, mustard, sea salt.

The Alkaline Diet Myth:

The soluble diet is also commonly referred to as the acid alkaline diet or alkaline ash diet.

It revolves around the premise that the food you consume has the potential to alter the acidity or alkalinity (the pH level) of your body.

How it Function:

When undergoing the process of metabolizing nutrients and extracting energy (calories) from them, one is effectively engaging in the combustion of food, albeit in a gradual and regulated manner.

When one burns sustenance, they indeed produce residual ashes, akin to the result of burning wood in a furnace.

Considering the circumstances, this residue can exhibit acidity, solubility, or neutrality... and proponents of this dietary approach assert that this residue can directly impact the alkalinity of your body.

In the event that one consumes food containing acidic ash, it leads to an increase in body acidity. In the event that one consumes food high in alkaline residue, it results in the alkalization of the body. The impartial remnants hold no consequence. Straightforward.

It is believed that the caustic embers render individuals vulnerable to disease and illness, whereas soluble slag is considered to be protective. Through the selection of highly soluble nourishments, one can effectively enhance their diet and promote better overall health.

Acidic residue leaving components in sustenance consist of protein, phosphate, and sulfur, whereas alkaline components include calcium, magnesium, and potassium.

Certain nutritional courses are regarded as acidic, alkaline, or neutral.

Acidic food items include meat, poultry, fish, dairy products, eggs, grains, and alcoholic beverages.

• Unbiased: Unprocessed fats, carbohydrates, and sweeteners. •

Neutral: Organic fats, starches, and sugars. • Impartial: Unrefined fats, carbohydrates, and sweeteners. • Objective: Untreated fats, starches, and sugars. • Fair: Raw fats, carbohydrates, and sweeteners. • Disinterested: Whole fats, starches, and sugars.

✓ Capable of dissolution: Fruits, nuts, vegetables

Dietary Restrictions and Allowances
The majority of agricultural produce, such as soybeans and tofu, along with select nuts, seeds, and vegetables, are considered soluble nutrient-rich foods, making them suitable for consumption.
Dairy products, eggs, meat, major cereal crops, as well as processed foods such as canned and packaged snacks, and convenient meals, belong to the acidic category and are prohibited.
Many literature pieces advocating for the fundamental dietary guidelines also

advise against the consumption of alcohol or caffeine.

Diet composition:
According to the traditional theory underlying this dietary approach, acid ash is generated by meat, poultry, cheese, fish, eggs, and grains.
Leafy vegetables, with the exception of cranberries, prunes, and plums, are responsible for the production of antacid fiery debris. Because the assignment of corrosive or soluble fiery debris relies on the residue left after combustion rather than the acidity of the food, it is important to note that foods typically considered acidic, such as citrus fruits, are actually regarded as alkaline-forming in this dietary context.

Why Is This Important?

When consuming acidic-forming food, our body must make a concerted effort to restore equilibrium to our blood pH. This is achieved by releasing highly soluble minerals, such as calcium, phosphorus, and magnesium, into our bloodstream.

If we do not consume an adequate amount of soluble framing nutrients, our body will necessitate extracting these essential minerals from our bones, teeth, and organs. This has the potential to compromise our secure infrastructure, induce fatigue, and render us susceptible to infections and diseases.

Some Tips:

Consume a diet comprising of 60-80% alkalizing foods and 20-40% acidifying foods.

To steer clear of corrosive-forming edibles, it is advisable to refrain from consuming fast-food burgers and processed meals. Instead, opt for more advantageous options such as legumes, cereals, and other fresh food sources. Pesticides possess a propensity for inducing corrosive effects on crops, thus it is advisable to opt for organic fruits and vegetables whenever feasible.

Important information to be aware of:" "Valuable knowledge to keep in mind:" "Crucial details to acquaint oneself with:" "Relevant points to acknowledge:" "Essential facts to understand:" "Significant matters to be mindful of:

The implementation of an ALKALINE DIET could prove to be highly beneficial in enhancing the effectiveness of specific types of chemotherapy medications.

A highly acidic diet creates an optimal environment for the proliferation of yeast and fungi. When transitioning to a diet of higher alkalinity, individuals may observe an increase in energy levels and a resolution of chronic yeast infections.

Final Verdict:
A soluble dietary approach emphasizes the consumption of alkaline foods, such as fruits and vegetables, as well as specific whole grains that have a low caloric density. Prominent examples of alkaline diet foods epitomize the delicate equilibrium between acidic and alkaline nourishment.

Why do certain foods pose challenges?

To address this query, let us initially contemplate the underlying factors that contribute to the occurrence of acid reflux ailment. The nourishment enters the gastric cavity by means of the esophagus. In the gastric cavity, the process of digestion commences as the food undergoes the action of digestive enzymes and hydrochloric acid that reside in the stomach. The sustenance persists confined within the abdominal cavity through the operation of valves located at both termini of the gastric organ. Owing to the acidic conditions prevailing within the stomach, occasional elevation in pressure may result in the opening of the valve. This leads to the migration of the stomach's acidic contents into the esophagus. This condition is commonly referred to as acid reflux.

It is evident that as the acidity level of the stomach increases, the pressure exerted on the lower esophageal sphincter valve also increases, thereby raising the likelihood of acid reflux. Therefore, in order to address the issue of acid reflux, it is advisable to refrain from consuming foods that promote the production of acid.

Recommended Dietary Restrictions for Acid Reflux Management

After discussing acidic foods, let us now enumerate specific food items falling under this category that can potentially induce symptoms of acid reflux. Red meat is an example of such food. Rather, consider selecting fish that offer exceptional nutritional value and promote overall well-being.

One should also cease the consumption of dairy products. This encompasses not just milk but also creams, cheeses, ice cream, milkshakes, and any other food item that utilizes dairy. In addition to lactose-based products, individuals with acid reflux are also advised against consuming chocolate. Consumption of food products such as pasta and macaroni should also be excluded from one's diet. Alternatively, whole grain bread can be utilized. Numerous individuals have reported alleviation of acid reflux symptoms through the consumption of low-fat yogurt. Fruits and vegetables typically have an alkaline nature and should be consumed in sufficient amounts. It is advisable to refrain from consuming tomatoes and tomato-based products. This encompasses tomato-based sauces and even preserved tomatoes in the form of pickles.

It is crucial to utilize minimal quantities of oil and spices during the cooking process to mitigate acid reflux. There exists a direct correlation between acid reflux and obesity. Individuals who possess a greater body mass are at an increased likelihood of experiencing gastroesophageal reflux disease. Therefore, it is advisable to also refrain from consuming foods that are high in carbohydrates and fat.

Selecting Appropriate Dietary Choices for Managing Acid Reflux

Selecting the appropriate dietary choices to alleviate acid reflux can present a challenge, particularly for individuals who are highly discerning about their dietary preferences. Where there is determination, there is always a solution. By employing a modicum of ingenuity and artistic flair, individuals can yet discover alternatives for their preferred culinary choices. For instance, rather than choosing a serving of ice cream for dessert, individuals may consider selecting a fruit salad paired with whipped low-fat yogurt.

Not all foods have the potential to induce acid reflux in all individuals. The condition fluctuates from individual to individual. While it is possible for certain individuals to experience acid reflux shortly after consuming a chocolate bar, others may not encounter such effects. It is essential to endeavor in observing whether a specific type of food is inducing acid reflux.

You may need to forgo indulging in your preferred hotdog or beef corn sandwich when managing the challenges associated with acid reflux. Opting for more nutritious cooking methods, such as baking and grilling, can also be advantageous. The process of frying has the potential to not only diminish the nutritional content of foods but also exacerbate symptoms of acid reflux.

However, fruits such as pineapple, banana, and apple are recognized for their ability to neutralize excessive stomach acid and mitigate acid reflux. Additionally, vegetables such as broccoli, cabbage, and cauliflower possess alkaline properties that aid in the prevention of acid reflux symptoms.

Despite the fact that individuals possess an understanding that maintaining a proper diet contributes to the preservation of youth and overall well-being, the majority are unacquainted with an appropriate dietary regimen that can effectively lead to a healthy physique. Alkaline meals are regarded as the optimal approach for maintaining a state of wellbeing, as they have the ability to modulate the body's pH levels and enhance various bodily functions such as digestion and metabolism. The ensuing passages will expound upon several advantages associated with choosing to adopt an alkaline diet.

• Alkaline meals encompass the ingestion of an assortment of vegetables, nuts, wheat grass, and barley grass. Almonds and tomatoes are included in this dietary regimen; nevertheless, the majority of health professionals recommend the consumption of barley grass and wheat grass due to the numerous additional advantages they provide. These meals provide essential nutrients to the body that facilitate the regulation of pH levels, thereby diminishing the likelihood of skin issues, cardiovascular conditions, and other health ailments. Numerous individuals who have chosen these meals have observed a decrease in skin complications, including imperfections and acne, within a remarkably short period of just two weeks.

• Alkaline meals are not associated with a passing trend in diets, thus individuals who choose these meals need not be concerned about adverse consequences once they cease adhering to the diet. Nevertheless, the majority of individuals who choose these meals tend to persist in consuming at least a portion of the suggested food items indefinitely, particularly due to the enduring advantages offered by recommended items like barley grass.

• Alkaline meals help to regulate the body's pH levels, and unlike processed food products, they do not result in sodium retention within the body. Contrary to the suggested dietary items, these recommended foods effectively purify the body and promote overall well-being. A considerable number of individuals who have chosen to adhere to this dietary regimen have also observed significant reduction in body weight and experienced various other advantages after following this diet for a few months. It should be emphasized that in order to fully reap the advantages of alkaline meals, it is imperative to adhere to this dietary regimen for a minimum duration of six months, if not longer, ideally extending up to a year or beyond.

• Alkaline meals offer enhanced levels of energy, thereby resulting in increased vitality and sustained vigor for individuals who consume such meals. These meals additionally offer a range of minerals and vitamins to the body, effectively counteracting acid imbalance. Given that alkaline foods are readily available, individuals with an inclination towards maintaining a healthy lifestyle can effortlessly achieve their objectives.

Understanding the Guidelines and Restrictions of the Alkaline Diet

The majority of the diets we are familiar with are designed with a focus on achieving weight reduction. Considering the global pursuit of attaining a leaner physique and improved appearance, it is evident that a substantial number of individuals are actively seeking diet strategies. The alkaline diet is similarly structured, with the added emphasis on fostering a lifestyle free from illnesses. Does it work? In order to comprehend this, it is crucial to acknowledge that the alkaline diet advocates for the consumption of alkaline foods. Consequently, there exist several guidelines to follow and precautions to take in one's diet, some of which can be quite extreme, particularly for individuals accustomed to a diet predominantly comprised of meat and dairy products. In this discourse, we shall delve into the concept of the alkaline diet and elucidate a comprehensive analysis of its recommended practices and cautionary measures.

The Dos:

The alkaline diet may be referred to as a natural diet due to its substantial inclusion of fruits and vegetables. Therefore, it is advisable that your dietary intake primarily comprises fruits and vegetables, as the majority of the available options are permissible. One may also consider incorporating various soy-based products, such as tofu and soybeans. Additional items that must be included in your inventory encompass several varieties of nuts, an assortment of seeds, as well as a selection of lentils and legumes. With regard to grains, there are certain limitations, which can be located through online sources. Certain specialists have advocated for the utilization of water fortified with essential vitamins. Essentially, this constitutes high-pH water that can potentially provide advantageous effects on the body similar to those offered by alkaline-promoting foods.

The Don\\\'ts:

If you are planning to adhere to the alkaline diet, the importance of the dos likely surpasses that of the don'ts. Prioritize the reduction of meat and dairy consumption in your diet as an initial step. It is also imperative to eliminate eggs and any types of canned, processed, and packaged food items from your diet, including chips, ready-made meals, and even popcorn. By consulting several literature sources pertaining to the alkaline diet, one will come to the realization that the consumption of alcohol is strictly prohibited as well. Furthermore, it is advised to reduce consumption of tea, coffee, and any other beverages that potentially contain caffeine.

Will I Lose Weight?

Now, that is a question frequently posed, primarily due to the fact that this is one of the diets that requires significant effort. The alkaline diet does not possess any miraculous properties. It does not guarantee immediate weight loss like the GM diet or similar diet plans. However, since it entails consuming a greater portion of fresh and wholesome foods, you can expect a substantial reduction in your body weight. In addition, reducing the consumption of processed food also yields a noteworthy impact. By consuming processed and unhealthy food, you are simultaneously restricting your sugar consumption, thereby adversely affecting the process of weight reduction.

Why The Alkaline Diet? The Benefits It Can Provide You

There has been considerable discussion regarding the alkaline diet, particularly in recent times. It appears that there is consistently an array of diets that gain prominence as the newest trend, yet this particular one has persistently remained one of the most favored choices. In addition, the objective of this dietary regimen is not solely to attain swift weight reduction, but rather to foster enduring wellness and vitality. This holds significance due to the fact that this attribute is uncommon among most other diets, which primarily focus on rapid weight loss at the expense of overall bodily wellbeing.

To adhere to the alkaline diet, it is essential to structure your meals with a primary focus on incorporating fresh fruits and vegetables. These are the food items that impart maximum nutritional benefits to the body and hence, should constitute the primary constituents of the diet. This particular dietary regimen has an extensive historical tenure, surpassing the longevity of virtually all other conventional diets. There are several specific reasons as to why an individual would find this dietary regimen beneficial. Individuals who possess a diminished amount of energy may experience a heightened sense of vitality and wakefulness following consistent adherence to the aforementioned practices for a span of several weeks.

Various studies have been conducted to evaluate the efficacy of the alkaline diet, and the findings consistently indicate its effectiveness. This holds particularly true when considering the fact that the majority of individuals adhere to the modified Western diet, characterized by its elevated content of fatty, sugary, and processed foods. It is essential to possess a comprehensive understanding of one's actions and avoid eliminating crucial food items that contribute to maintaining the overall well-being of the body. Individuals afflicted with renal issues are advised to refrain from following this dietary regimen, as it has the potential to exacerbate their condition.

If you meet the suitability criteria for adhering to this dietary plan, it will be necessary for you to systematically eliminate all unhealthy food items from your pantry. The abundance of unhealthy food present in people's homes often catches them off guard. This is equally significant as it will aid in avoiding temptation. If you truly desire to adhere to the alkaline diet, it is imperative to eliminate all forms of temptation and wholeheartedly dedicate yourself to this cause.

In terms of outcomes, you will observe them nearly instantaneously when adhering to the alkaline diet. The outcomes are so favorable that the majority of individuals discover it conveniently manageable to adhere to the diet once they become aware of the initial indication of any alteration. Ensure regular physical activity is incorporated into your routine alongside your alkaline diet to optimize outcomes. It undeniably provides numerous advantages over other diets available today.

2: Acidosis

At this juncture, you might be pondering upon the measures you can take if you are burdened with a condition in which an acidic state of your body has led to health complications. You are required to comprehend the definition of acidosis, its impact on the human body, as well as the strategies for overcoming it.

What is acidosis?

Acidosis refers to the condition in which the body contains an abundance of acid. It entails surpassing a specific threshold of acidity within the bloodstream and bodily tissues. The blood pH level within the arterial vessels is expected to be 7.35. In the event that it decreases below said threshold, individuals may potentially experience low-grade or chronic acidosis, thereby having an impact on the overall cellular functionality throughout the body. Acidosis has an impact on cellular activities and their corresponding functions.

The consumption of processed foods with high caloric content constitutes a predominant component of contemporary dietary patterns. Our bodies lack the ability to efficiently metabolize these foods; consequently, diseases such as cancer, diabetes, heart conditions, and other health ailments have become increasingly prevalent. In order to achieve a well-being that promotes longevity and vitality, it is imperative to adhere to the alkaline diet, characterized by an emphasis on consuming foods with high alkaline content and minimizing the intake of acid-forming foods. This is the impact they exert on the human physique.

An acidogenic diet consists of food items whose consumption leads to the development of acidic indigestion within the body, ultimately resulting in the occurrence of the acidosis condition.

"The etiological factors contributing to acidosis are:

eating acid-forming foods

medications

chemical toxins

immune system reactions

stress

tobacco intake

alcohol intake

health conditions such as diabetes

The primary cause of acidosis can be attributed to a dietary pattern characterized by the consumption of acid-forming foods and a lower intake of alkaline-promoting foods. Indeed, approximately 95% of all instances of acidosis can be attributed to the ingestion of diets that promote the production of acidic substances. The physiological processes of body cells and tissues, organs, as well as the digestive and excretory systems, can be influenced by deviations in pH levels. It is imperative to monitor and regulate pH levels in order to mitigate potential health complications.

Currently, individuals exhibit a greater preference for convenience as opposed to prioritizing their well-being. They consume fast foods and processed foods abundant in refined sugar and devoid of nutritional value, neglecting to prioritize their health in the appropriate manner.

French fries, burgers, doughnuts, soft drinks, and sandwiches are readily available for selection at a variety of establishments such as esteemed hotels, renowned restaurants, charming cafés, well-stocked grocery stores, and convenient convenience stores that are abundantly dispersed throughout the region.

The majority of these food items and dietary regimens contain devoid calories that fail to provide the body with the necessary nutrients it requires. Nevertheless, we continue to partake in their consumption on a daily basis. Furthermore, we go as far as stocking our refrigerators with these comestibles and libations, ensuring convenient access whenever they are desired.

As individuals consume meals on the go and engage in the combination of incompatible foodstuffs, they frequently encounter indigestion, thereby resulting in the persistent emergence of acidosis, which exerts adverse effects on cellular functioning. The cells progressively lose their ability to carry out their typical physiological functions, which subsequently leads to the onset of various afflictions and medical conditions. They commence the process of counterbalancing the surplus acids and eliminating them from the body to avert their infiltration into critical organs, thereby imposing a burden on the same.

Cells under stress are unable to adequately carry out their intended functions, underscoring the importance of promptly adopting an alkaline diet.

Acidosis fosters an environment that is detrimental to the cellular structures, internal organs, muscular system, skeletal framework, and articulations.

The cells experience a depletion in their energy reserves, thereby compromising the efficacy of the immune system and leading to the onset of various medical ailments such as cancer, obesity, as well as skeletal disorders like arthritis and osteoporosis. These aforementioned health conditions have the potential to manifest abruptly or gradually emerge over time, coinciding with an increased level of acidity within the body.

In circumstances where cells manifest a low pH and experience oxygen deprivation, it gives rise to the proliferation of bacteria, viruses, molds, and fungi within or upon the organism. Our physiological well-being necessitates the maintenance of an optimal alkaline environment within our bodies. To uphold an optimal pH equilibrium, it is necessary to consume a diet consisting of 80% alkalizing foods and beverages while limiting acid-forming ones to 20%.

The majority of experts suggest maintaining a dietary balance between 60% to 80% alkaline foods. The consumption of nutritionally void calories results in the depletion of cellular energy required for the process of detoxification. This depletes the body of its vitality and vitality.

Effects of acidosis

Food items are regarded as acidogenic due to their impact on the human body and the residual acidity they generate upon digestion. Therefore, acidic citrus foods such as grapefruits, lemons, and limes are considered to be foods that promote alkalinity.

Acidic food items include meat, eggs, sugar, wheat flour products, dairy products like milk, poultry, eggs, cheese, caffeine, grains, and fruits such as plums, cranberries, prunes, and soft drinks.

The consumption of a dietary pattern characterized by an abundance of low alkaline and high acidic foods fosters an environment conducive to the proliferation of diseases. Cancer, stroke, cardiovascular illnesses, renal complications, inadequate nutrient intake, and cognitive decline flourish in an acidic milieu, which leads to an acidic pH level and insufficient oxygen supply. The occurrence of acidosis prompts the formation of cancerous cells as well as other diseased cells.

There has been considerable discussion surrounding the appropriate daily water intake, yet the authoritative guideline from the Department of Health stipulates a recommended quantity of 1.2 liters per day.

There exists a commonly mentioned value suggesting that we should intake 2.5 liters on a daily basis. However, this value is somewhat ambiguous, as it pertains to the overall amount of fluid lost per day and our corresponding replenishment needs.

It is not necessarily mandated that we adhere to the complete replacement obligation in the context of hydration, since roughly 1 liter of fluid can be derived from the consumption of food and an additional 0.3 liters from physiological reactions. This is the origin of the 1.2 liters per day statistic. In order to provide a contextual framework, it can be stated that the aforementioned quantity is equivalent to 8 glasses of water, provided that each individual glass contains a volume of 150ml.

The health advantages associated with the consumption of water extend beyond commonly acknowledged assertions. Inadequate hydration can lead to muscle fatigue, as muscle tissue undergoes contraction and atrophy due to an imbalance in the levels of fluid and electrolytes. Furthermore, there is substantiating evidence that adequate hydration is conducive to the promotion of optimal skin health.

Proper hydration is advantageous for the optimal functioning of your kidneys, as it reduces the burden on their function in waste filtration and processing. Sufficient water availability additionally facilitates the smooth passage of waste through the system, as it prevents the kidneys from needing to retain fluid in the urine.

Numerous additional assertions prevail regarding the benefits of adequate hydration for the human body. Dehydration has been associated with heartburn, arthritis, back pain, angina, migraines, colitis, asthma, and hypertension, among other conditions.

The fact of the matter is that the human body is a machine that operates on a foundation of water. Water functions as both a lubricant and a source of fuel. If the machine does not have an intake mechanism that sufficiently makes up for the natural losses it undergoes on a daily basis, it will be unable to operate effectively and will eventually experience a breakdown.

Alkaline Water

Alkaline potable water encompasses essential nutrients such as magnesium, calcium, salt, and potassium in a readily digestible form, aiding the body's nourishment. Ionic technology modifies the molecular composition of water into only 5 or 6 constituents per cluster, allowing convenient accessibility to the cellular structure.

The specific pH level of this drinking water facilitates expedited hydration of the body and contributes to regulating body temperature for enhanced well-being.

In selected regions where there is an inadequacy of calcium in the water, it is possible to introduce calcium supplements to the water ionizer, which will then facilitate the incorporation of calcium into the ionized water to meet the body's calcium requirements.

The electrolysis process implemented by the drinking water ionizer facilitates the reorganization of the naturally occurring minerals in the billed water, resulting in their enhanced bioavailability for the human body. Ionized drinking water can effectively diminish toxins, enhance vitality levels, promote a balanced alkaline/acidic ratio, hydrate tissues, thereby fostering a robust bodily state accompanied by increased vitality.

Symptoms such as fatigue and unease are indicative of an excessive level of acidity in the body. The consumption of additional ionized water may prove beneficial in such circumstances.

Upon consuming alkaline water, we are partaking in a potent and entirely organic antioxidant that revitalizes the body.

Consuming water with optimal pH levels aids in the absorption of nutrients, provides protection against viral and bacterial infections, and facilitates the elimination of waste products.

1. Alkaline potable water contains essential calcium, magnesium, sodium, and potassium minerals that are readily absorbed by the body.

Cancer malignancy does not thrive in an environment that is abundant in oxygen and maintains alkalinity.

Alkaline water facilitates equilibrium in pH levels to enhance overall well-being.

2. Ionized alkaline water is comprised of smaller compound clusters that aid the body in effectively processing larger quantities of water and maintaining optimal hydration.

3. Employing alkaline water to dilute your juices from concentrate will result in a more enhanced taste profile; this applies equally to coffee and tea.

The natural structure and color of fruits and vegetables remain intact when they are cooked using alkaline water.

The grain is expected to become more buoyant following its immersion in alkaline water and subsequent boiling.

Alkaline ionized water facilitates weight loss and suppresses appetite during dietary regimens.

Consume a minimum of 8-10 fluid ounces of water on a daily basis.

The Significance of Alkaline for Human Physiology

In order to maintain optimal bodily health, it is imperative that the equilibrium between alkaline and acid levels is upheld, a metric quantified by the pH value within the system. The pH values span from 0 to 14, with 7 being considered as neutral. A value below 7 is regarded as acidic." "In the realm of acidity, any value lower than 7 is considered acidic." "Values below 7 are classified as acidic." "When the value falls below 7, it is deemed as acidic." "In the context of acidity, any value less than 7 is coined as acidic. Processed foods, including meat products, confectioneries, and certain sweetened beverages, tend to induce a substantial acid load on the human body.

Acidosis, characterized by elevated levels of acidity in the bloodstream and cells, serves as a prevalent indicator of various diseases afflicting a significant number of individuals. Several health practitioners assert that acidosis is accountable for the severe ailments experienced by numerous individuals in the present era.

An alkaline or alkaline diet, typically inherent in our biological system, serves to counteract the elevated acidity within the body, thereby attaining a state of equilibrium. This constitutes the primary role of the alkaline within the human body. However, the alkaline levels in the body are rapidly depleted due to the elevated concentration of acidic substances it must neutralize, and there is an insufficient ingestion of alkaline food to replenish the depletion of alkaline substances.

Attaining an Equilibrium of Alkaline and Acid Levels to Promote Optimal Health

As mentioned earlier, acidosis gives rise to numerous health-related complications. When an excessive amount of acid permeates our system, it causes the disintegration of cells and organs if not effectively neutralized. In order to mitigate this, it is imperative to ensure that a well-balanced pH level is upheld.

The determination of elevated alkalinity levels in our bodies can be easily conducted for diagnostic purposes. This is accomplished by means of pH strips, which can be obtained from any reputable pharmacy. There exist two distinct categories of strips, one meant for saliva analysis and the other designed for urine testing.

In general, the pH level of saliva can be assessed using a strip to determine the acidity level produced by the body. Ideally, the pH values should fall within the range of 6.5 to 7.5 throughout the course of the day. A urinary pH level strip will indicate the acidity level; a typical measurement should fall within the range of 6.0 to 6.5 in the morning and between 6.5 and 7.0 at night.

Excessively Acidic Conditions Can Be Detrimental to the Human Body.

If one frequently experiences fatigue, headaches, and recurrent instances of the common cold and flu, these symptoms are indicative of an elevated acidity level within the body. The presence of acidosis within the human body not only hampers the customary ailments recognized within medical research, but also contributes to the development of various other disorders that may be experienced, arising from an elevated accumulation of acidic compounds within the system.

Depression, elevated acidity, gastric ulcers, parched skin, acne, and excessive body weight are some of the manifestations associated with an excessive degree of acidity within our physiological system. In addition to the aforementioned conditions, there exist several other significant ailments such as arthritis, osteoporosis, bronchitis, recurrent infections, and cardiovascular diseases.

Despite the administration of medications, the symptoms may be masked, persisting to exert an impact on your well-being due to the incomplete eradication of the underlying issue. Increasing the dosage of medication will merely exacerbate the issue, as the administration of additional anti-inflammatory drugs will contribute to the acidic imbalance in the body.

Chapter 4

Application of Alkaline Diets in the Management of Diabetes

The sustenance of the body's alkaline levels guarantees the optimal functioning of the body. Despite the fact that the end products of metabolism are frequently acidic, the body inherently maintains an alkaline state.

The internal milieu or environment of the human body is characterized by a mild alkaline state, thereby necessitating the adoption of a diet that similarly maintains a slightly alkaline nature. The metabolic processes of the body necessitate an alkaline milieu for optimal efficiency. The human organism consists of billions of cells, and each bodily function occurs on the cellular scale. The cellular structures possess a minor alkaline state and necessitate continual alkalinity for proper function and overall preservation of well-being and vitality.

Acidosis arises from the overconsumption of acid-generating foods and inadequate intake of alkaline-forming foods, leading to the exacerbation of acid intoxication within the body. Over time, the accumulation of toxic waste and the secretion of acidic waste from the body will result in the onset of acidosis. The condition known as acidosis is synonymous with excessive acidity within the human body.

The occurrence of acidosis has been linked to the emergence of degenerative chronic ailments, particularly diabetes, along with other conditions such as cancer, arthritis, and heart diseases. Acidosis gradually undermines the essential bodily functions, particularly in the absence of timely remedial measures. Moreover, it has been identified that acidosis serves as a primary factor in the process of human aging.

Individuals afflicted with diabetes can enhance their general physical well-being by adhering to alkaline diets. The primary concern for individuals with diabetes lies in addressing acidosis resulting from elevated blood glucose levels. By adhering to an alkaline diet, individuals with diabetes will be able to effectively address metabolic concerns and enhance the balance of their physiological pH levels. The immune system is an additional aspect that will be targeted and enhanced through the implementation of an alkaline diet.

Alkaline diets can facilitate improved glycemic control in individuals with diabetes. In addition, alkaline diets can offer the benefit of assisting individuals with diabetes in mitigating and managing optimal body weight, while effectively mitigating the likelihood of cardiovascular diseases by actively regulating low cholesterol levels.

In essence, the alkaline diets facilitate improved diabetes management for patients. Consequently, individuals with diabetes can effectively mitigate their susceptibility to degenerative ailments associated with the condition. The alkaline diet effectively promotes improved well-being and significantly enhances the life expectancy of individuals with diabetes.

The prevailing guideline for individuals with diabetes seeking to initiate and adhere to an alkaline diet is to ensure that their daily dietary choices consist of at least 80 percent alkaline-forming foods, while limiting acidifying foods to no more than 20 percent of their overall food intake. In order to gain a more comprehensive grasp of this rule, it is important to note that food items with higher levels of alkalinity are considered more beneficial, whereas those that are more acidifying tend to have adverse effects on the human body, particularly for individuals with diabetes.

For individuals seeking to employ alkaline diets for diabetes management, a Diabetics Acid-Alkaline Food Chart has been developed in collaboration with the American Diabetes Association and the University of Sydney. The chart has classified alkalizing foods into six distinct groups based on their glycemic index (GI). The list considers the highest quality foods as well as the lowest quality foods when adhering to an alkalizing diet.

1. Foods with a glycemic index (GI) of approximately zero that have alkalizing properties. These food items constitute a selection of the finest choices that should be incorporated into an alkaline-promoting dietary regimen. These are dietary options that are permissible for individuals with diabetes to consume without restriction. They are:

The following items are included in the list: avocados, asparagus, beans, green tea, beets, broccoli, cabbage, flax-seed oil, carob, celery, lemon water, raw spinach, lettuce, vegetable juices, mushrooms, herbal teas, squash, okra, cauliflower, garlic, onions, lemons, limes, goat cheese, olive oil, parsley, stevia, ginger tea, canola oil, zucchini.

2. Food items with a glycemic index (GI) of 55 or below that possess alkalizing properties. Individuals with diabetes should consume these items in moderation due to their slightly elevated glycemic index. Some illustrations of consumable items falling within this particular classification include:

The list comprises the following items: almonds, barley grass, carrots, olives, soybeans, bananas, cherries, oranges, peaches, pears, mangoes, peas, kiwi, papayas, berries, Brazil nut, chestnuts, hazelnuts, coconut, quinoa, lentils, soy milk, apples, soy cheese, grapefruit, goat milk, tomatoes, breast milk, fresh corn, wild rice, raw honey, sweet potato, and whey.

3. Utilizing food items with a glycemic index (GI) close to negligible levels to induce acidification. Patients diagnosed with diabetes should exercise caution

when consuming foods in this particular category due to the acidogenic properties of such foods.

Artificial sweeteners, rhubarb, pork, liver, beef, venison, cold water fish, turkey, eggs, butter, cottage cheese, corn oil, margarine, sunflower oil, lard, wine, cheese, beer, coffee, buttermilk, cocoa, chicken, tea, lamb, mayonnaise, oysters, molasses, shellfish, mustard, cooked spinach, vinegar. Artificial sweeteners, rhubarb, pork, liver, beef, venison, cold water fish, turkey, eggs, butter, cottage cheese, corn oil, margarine, sunflower oil, lard, wine, cheese, beer, coffee, buttermilk, cocoa, chicken, tea, lamb, mayonnaise, oysters, molasses, shellfish, mustard, cooked spinach, vinegar.

4. Consuming acidic food items that have a glycemic index (GI) value of 55 or below. It is advisable to consume the foods with moderation, taking into

account their tendency to promote acid formation and their high glycemic index. The foods are:

The following items are included: lima beans, kidney beans, blueberries, sour cherries, plums, sprouted wheat bread, corn, oats/rye, whole wheat/rye bread, wheat, peanuts, cashews, pecans, pistachios, sunflower seeds, sesame, walnuts, yogurt, pasta/pastries, cream, brown rice, raw milk, prunes, custard, cranberries, homogenized milk, pinto beans, ice cream, navy beans, and chocolate.

5. Food items that promote alkalinity with a glycemic index (GI) of 56 or higher. It is advised for individuals with diabetes to steer clear of these food items on account of their elevated glycemic index. Some illustrations of these edibles include:

The following items are included: Amaranth, beetroot, turnip, raw sugar, tofu, figs, dates, grapes or raisins, melons, watermelon, rice syrup, potato with skins, maple syrup, pineapple, and millet.

6. Food items that have a glycemic index (GI) score of 56 or higher and contribute to acid production. The vast majority of the food items falling under this particular category predominantly consist of carbohydrates, which possess pronounced acidity and exhibit a remarkably high glycemic index. It is imperative for individuals with diabetes to abstain entirely from including them in their dietary consumption.

Ultimately, it can be concluded that fresh vegetables and grasses possess noteworthy properties that make them highly effective in combating yeast and fungal infections. Green grasses, such as barley or wheat grass, exhibit remarkable characteristics including being exceptionally low in calories and sugar content, while also boasting an abundant array of essential nutrients. They are well-suited for individuals who have a strong desire to establish a solid basis for their well-being, both in the present and for the foreseeable future.

Frequently Inquired Queries regarding the Dietary Regimen

Does the process of cooking have an impact on the pH levels and acid-alkaline balance of food?

Response: No, it does not. The acidity or alkalinity of food remains unchanged due to the lack of any significant alteration in their chemical composition. The process of cooking could potentially alter the structure of the food, but it does not have an impact on the pH level.

Inquiry 2: What is the correlation between alkaline food and the occurrence of acid reflux?

Response: Incorporating alkaline foods into your diet can effectively mitigate the intensity of acid reflux symptoms by ensuring optimal pH balance in the gastrointestinal tract. However, it should be noted that a diet exclusively designed for managing acid reflux varies from the alkaline diet expounded upon within the pages of this book.

Inquiry 3: In what manner does the consumption of alkaline food contribute to weight loss?

Response: In order to transition to a more alkaline diet, it is essential to exclude certain food items such as sugars, complex carbohydrates, legumes, and cereal grains. Excluding these food varieties from your diet can facilitate weight loss.

Classifying food items: foods that produce acidity and foods that produce alkalinity.

Acid-forming foods

When individuals consume acidic food, the residual byproduct of the metabolic process manifests as acidic waste. Subsequently, this waste necessitates traversing the body, inducing an acidic internal environment that can manifest as lethargy or even the manifestation of various ailments. Opting for the consumption of alkaline foods generates the beneficial alkaline residue, which bestows numerous advantages upon the body.

What are the types of naturally acidic foods, specifically those that result in an acidic residue within the body upon metabolism? Those foods include:

Any food that is rich in sodium

Processed foods

Fast foods

Preserved meats such as deli meats

Breakfast cereals that are manufactured and packaged in boxes

Beverages that are enriched with caffeine, such as coffee

Most grain products

Rice varieties available include white, brown, and basmati.

Cheese

Pasta

Wheat germ

Alcoholic drinks

All types of meat, including beef, pork, lamb, fish, and chicken

Mustard

Ketchup

Soy sauce

Popcorn

Mayonnaise

White vinegar

Nutmeg

Tobacco

Cornmeal, rye

Colas

Sweetened yogurt

Refined table salt

White bread

White pasta

Walnuts, Peanuts

All dairy products

Eggs

Artificial sweeteners

Animal meats sourced from animals that have not been raised on a grass-fed diet.

Additives such as preservatives and food coloring

Seafood

Consuming diets high in acid-forming foods can enhance the excretion of calcium from the bones, leading to subsequent loss of calcium through urination. This would ultimately result in a reduction in bone density and potentially give rise to ailments such as osteoporosis.

GERD (Gastroesophageal reflux disease) is a persistent medical disorder characterized by the retrograde movement of gastric acid from the stomach, regurgitating it into the esophagus. Acidic food items frequently exacerbate the underlying factors of acid reflux by inducing loosening of the muscular band responsible for retaining acid within the stomach.

Foods with higher levels of acidity result in a decrease in the pH levels of urine. The organism is exerting optimal effort to expel surplus acid waste from the system via the urinary excretion process. This surplus will ultimately result in augmented occurrence of renal calculi and other ailments and disorders affecting the kidneys and urinary system.

Individuals who consume diets that consist primarily of acidic foods experience a higher prevalence of persistent muscular and joint pain and inflammation. The surplus of acid within the body has been scientifically associated with the development of chronic back pain, migraines, and muscle spasms.

Foods characterized by acidity and a low pH have the capacity to readily reduce the overall pH level in the human body.

The consumption of these foods can contribute to the onset of a multitude of conditions and diseases, making it a prudent choice to eliminate them from one's diet. By incorporating these practices and incorporating the recommended alkaline foods into your diet, you will experience a notable improvement in your well-being and initiate the initial stride towards cultivating a healthier way of living.

Alkaline-forming foods

Presented herein are several dietary options that align with the principles of the alkaline diet, elucidating the benefits they confer upon the body.

Fruits are included in the alkaline diet due to their alkaline properties and their ability to alleviate the body's chemistry and return it to a more alkaline state.

The majority of fruits contain substantial amounts of vitamins and minerals that support the development of an alkaline environment within the body.

Magnesium and potassium are essential minerals that play a crucial role in maintaining the body's acid-base balance. These minerals can be sourced from a variety of fruits including apples, avocados, bananas, cantaloupes, coconuts, grapefruits, grapes, honeydews, lemons, peaches, pineapples, plums, pumpkins, raisins, raspberries, and strawberries. Magnesium facilitates the augmentation of alkalinity within the body by providing energy to the muscular system. When the muscles experience an insufficient supply of energy, they undergo a metabolic process leading to the production of lactic acid, consequently altering the body's pH to an acidic state. Potassium also functions to maintain muscular strength, particularly pertaining to the cardiac and pulmonary muscles. The respiratory system functions to maintain an alkaline pH level by eliminating acidic toxins from the body through exhalation.

Vegetables are an additional crucial element that will facilitate the maintenance of pH equilibrium within the body, resulting in enhanced alkalinity. Vegetables serve as an additional viable reservoir of both potassium and magnesium, essential for facilitating optimal muscular performance as well as facilitating effective waste elimination by the heart and lungs. Artichokes, potatoes, bean sprouts, beets, bell peppers, broccoli, Brussel sprouts, cabbage, cauliflower, cucumbers, greens, kale, leeks, spinach, squash, sweet potatoes, yams, and zucchini all contain ample amounts of potassium and magnesium.

Dietary fiber assumes a significant role in promoting bodily health and mitigating body acidity. Fiber is an indigestible carbohydrate, unlike most carbohydrates that can undergo digestion to form sugar molecules within the bloodstream. Although some fiber is present in various fruits and vegetables, the greatest concentrations of fiber can be found in apples, apricots, berries, grapes, oranges, peaches, plums, raisins, artichokes, beets, celery, greens, lettuce, potatoes, and tomatoes. Fiber is also present in dried legumes such as pinto beans, navy beans, and kidney beans, as well as in various types of seeds like pumpkin seeds, sesame seeds, and chia seeds.

Alkaline water also constitutes a pivotal element within the framework of the alkaline diet. Alkaline water consists of a multitude of minerals, encompassing magnesium, potassium, and calcium.

Alkaline water demonstrates a reduced acid content relative to conventional tap water, thereby facilitating the process of counteracting acidic substances within the bloodstream. Furthermore, alkaline water can facilitate optimal metabolic functions within the body, thereby enhancing the body's utilization of essential vitamins and minerals. This, in turn, naturally promotes enhanced performance and improved overall well-being.

Given that the human body is predominantly composed of water, this particular substance holds significant importance within the context of human physiology. Alkaline water, characterized by an elevated pH level, contains a greater concentration of essential minerals crucial for maintaining optimum human health. Exclusive consumption of alkaline water has been found to aid in various aspects, such as the facilitation of cancer cell proliferation, facilitation of general weight reduction, detoxification of the body, facilitation of hydration, enhancement of skin health and appearance, as well as reinforcement of immune system functionality. Finally, alkaline water contributes to colon cleansing and serves as a preventive measure or decelerator for the general aging process.

In instances of excessive acidity within the body, it will utilize all accessible vitamins and minerals to facilitate the restoration of pH equilibrium. Therefore, an elevated concentration of acid within the body can result in a decrease in skeletal muscle mass, an elevation in adipose tissue accumulation, a reduction in essential growth-related hormone levels, and the formation of renal calculi.

Breakfast Omelette with Turmeric in Accordance with the Alkaline Diet

INGREDIENTS:

- 1 spring onion, finely sliced
- ¼ courgette, grated
- 1 tbsp. chopped parsley
- 3 organic eggs
- 2cm of fresh turmeric, finely grated
- Pinch of Himalayan salt
- 1 tbsp. sunflower oil

INSTRUCTIONS:

•Combine the eggs, grated turmeric, and salt in a bowl while vigorously stirring.

• Preheat a non-stick skillet and evenly distribute sunflower oil.

• Carefully transfer the egg mixture onto the pan, ensuring an even distribution, and garnish with the courgette, spring onion, and parsley.

• Cook for a duration of 3-4 minutes until the periphery is cooked while ensuring that the center achieves the desired consistency and avoids excessive liquidity.

• Carefully invert the egg with the spatula and proceed to cook it on the opposite side.

• Accompany the main dish with a side of salad and toast.

Alkaline Foods vs. Acidic Foods

In this discourse, I shall delineate the disparity that exists between Alkaline foods and Acidic foods, in addition to describing their reciprocal relationship. To begin with, it should be noted that the categorization of foods as acidic or alkaline is not solely based on one's perception or taste. While one might assume that a lemon is acidic due to its bitter taste, the classification of foods as alkaline or acidic is determined by the physiological processes occurring in the kidneys. Upon the arrival of nutrients in your kidneys, they generate either an increased amount of ammonium, classified as acidic, or they generate an augmented quantity of bicarbonate, categorized as alkaline. Scientists have developed a methodology for quantifying and evaluating the acid load present in foods, thereby enabling the measurement and assessment of their composition. This evaluative metric is known as PRAL, an acronym denoting Potential Renal Acid Load.

In illustration, it should be noted that grains, meat, fish, and eggs demonstrate an acidic nature and yield a positive PRAL score; conversely, fruits and vegetables exhibit an alkaline nature and yield a negative PRAL score.

Excessive consumption of acidic foods is associated with the risk of developing osteoporosis, as the body tends to extract minerals from the bones in order to maintain optimal pH levels.

Our objective with this dietary plan is to achieve a distribution of 80% and 20%. Comprising 80 percent alkaline foods, along with a remaining 20 percent allocation for non-processed or sugary foods. The proportion of foods that fall into this category would be comprised of 20 percent, including meats, fish, poultry, eggs, and similar items.

Similar to numerous dietary plans, the Alkaline diet primarily comprises an assortment of fruits and vegetables, exemplifying the finest options that include:

Some examples include raisins, dates, mushrooms, citrus fruits, tomatoes, spinach, celery, and cabbage, among others.

Raw foods are inherently superior to cooked foods; it is advisable to incorporate a significant portion of your dietary intake in its uncooked form. As it has been postulated to possess biogenic properties, bestowing vitality. When foods are subjected to cooking, the minerals responsible for maintaining alkalinity within your body are actually diminished. However, you still retain the regular benefits of vitamins.

One highly effective approach to augmenting the quantity of raw food consumption involves juicing, thereby enabling the reduction of overall intake to a mere one or two servings per day. Additionally, your body will receive an influx of essential nutrients and vitamins as a result of the concentrated formulation. Legumes and nuts offer equally favorable alternatives; noteworthy examples include almonds, green beans, lima beans, and walnuts. Green beverages or supplements, comprising powdered green vegetables and grasses, are rich in alkaline-forming foods, such as chlorophyll, which possesses a molecular structure closely resembling that of human blood.

Acidic foods or foods with an anti-alkaline nature exhibit substantial diversity and form a significant portion of the typical individual's dietary intake. Processed foods are largely to blame due to their elevated levels of sodium chloride, more commonly recognized as table salt. Excessive consumption of this can result in the blockage of arteries, causing constriction of blood vessels and the generation of heightened acidity.

"Now, let us examine Acidic and Anti-Alkaline Foods:

Processed cereals e.g. cornflakes.

Milk, in addition to inducing high levels of acidity within the body, also contains carbohydrates, which is a common characteristic of dairy products that are rich in calcium. To counterbalance this, it is advisable to consume ample quantities of leafy vegetables or extract the juices from leafy greens such as kale, spinach, and the like.

Regardless of whether whole wheat products are consumed or not, they uniformly lead to heightened acidity within the body. According to surveys, the majority of plant-based food consumed by Americans is in the form of processed corn or wheat.

Eggs, lentils, soft drinks, and coffee are all classified as highly acidic food items. Additionally, peanuts, walnuts, pasta, packaged grain, and bread are examples of food items that possess a substantial PRAL rating, indicating their high acidity content.

In addition to the consumption of certain foods, there exist additional factors that can contribute to elevated acidity levels. These include excessive intake of alcohol and drugs (including prescription medications), high levels of caffeine consumption, the presence of artificial sweeteners, heightened stress levels, and the ingestion of excessive amounts of animal meats and hormones derived from food sources. For example, products that pertain to health and beauty. While this inventory may not be exhaustive, it demonstrates that exposure to diverse factors can contribute to the accumulation of excessive acidity within the human organism.

If you perceive an imbalance in your diet or have not experienced satisfactory results from conventional treatments for a certain ailment, it may be prudent to contemplate adopting the Alkaline diet in order to mitigate the potential for enduring further adverse effects. As a result of a heightened consumption of Alkaline foods and limited contact with Acidic foods or substances that induce Acidic symptoms, you will begin to experience the advantages, even within a brief period of time. In the majority of instances, not only will you be negating the acidity in your physique, but you will also be subjecting your system to substantial quantities of indispensable nutrients. It is imperative to sustain this as a long-term alteration to one's lifestyle, lest the acidic PH levels lead to undesirable symptoms, illnesses, or diminished longevity. Therefore, it is imperative to effectuate this change for the better, as it will yield advantageous outcomes in the long run.

The pH of fluid around the cells is controlled by the renal system (kidneys). Whereas the respiratory system rapidly undergoes alterations to regulate pH levels, the renal system may require several days to respond to a pH shift and establish the necessary regulatory mechanisms. The renal system responds to discrepancies in the pH level by adjusting the secretion of acid into the bloodstream, accordingly to maintain equilibrium.

The human body consistently undergoes modifications and adaptations to maintain equilibrium in the pH levels across its different systems. The human body performs these functions instinctively as a result of neurologically transmitted signals between the brain and various physiological systems. The primary mechanism employed by the body to regulate acid levels is respiration, though the body also eliminates acid through urine, the integumentary system, and any alternative means to maintain an optimal blood pH. Therefore, in the situation where the body possesses the appropriate quantity of base yet an excessive amount of acid, the pH level is rendered acidic. If the body maintains an appropriate acid level while exhibiting an excess of base, it can be deemed alkaline.

Blood, saliva, and urine would exhibit distinctive variations in their pH levels. This disparity stems from the diverse physiological roles that these fluid-containing systems play within the human organism. While the coordination of numerous systems is essential for maintaining the body's optimal functioning, each system possesses distinctive autonomous functions that necessitate specific pH levels.

The standard pH range for the bloodstream is between 7.35 and 7.45. Blood exhibits a natural tendency towards slight alkalinity. In the event that the pH level in the bloodstream descends below 7.35, the blood undergoes excessive acidity, resulting in the gradual degradation of red blood cells. The kidneys and the lungs are the two primary organs that contribute significantly to the maintenance of the blood stream's pH equilibrium. The respiratory system employs the act of respiration to eliminate carbon dioxide (CO_2) through exhalation. The kidneys facilitate the removal of acid from the bloodstream via the process of urine formation. There exist multiple factors that can instigate fluctuations in the pH level of the blood. If the blood pH surpasses its designated range, an alkalotic condition is present within the body. The presence of an ailment can induce a temporary elevation in the blood pH level. In certain instances, specific food items can cause an elevation in the alkalinity of the pH levels in the bloodstream. Merely undergoing excessive fluid loss from the body can lead to an alteration in the blood pH equilibrium. Fluid loss can occur as a consequence of gastrointestinal issues such as diarrhea and vomiting, as well as excessive sweating. Certain medications, such as diuretics, have the potential to induce excessive urination, thereby resulting in elevated blood pH levels. In order to mitigate the consequences of an excessive loss of fluids, it is imperative to replenish both the actual fluid and the electrolytes that were depleted during the aforementioned procedure. Electrolytes consist of essential minerals and salts present in the body, namely potassium and sodium. Consuming a small amount of a sports beverage can aid in replenishing depleted electrolyte levels. When the kidneys fail to expel alkaline substances adequately via the urine, it can result in an elevation of blood pH as a consequence of renal issues.

The inherent pH range of saliva is between 6.2 and 7.6. The act of consuming beverages or food elicits an immediate alteration in the saliva's pH level as the body initiates the process of digestion. The gum and tooth health is directly impacted by the pH level in the oral cavity. The sole method of maintaining pH levels within a desired range is by monitoring and managing the intake of food. Maintaining a meticulous balance in the pH of the oral cavity will additionally contribute to the mitigation of oral bacteria, thereby diminishing the susceptibility to dental caries, periodontal disease, and cavities. The sugars present in food provide nourishment for the bacteria that naturally inhabit the oral cavity of humans. Certain food items such as bread, pasta, carbonated beverages, and confectioneries facilitate the nourishment of oral bacteria, thus promoting increased production of lactic acid, which directly contributes to the occurrence of dental decay. The lactic acid actively breaks down the dental plaque that accumulates on sound teeth. Although it is imperative to undergo routine plaque removal, it is important to note that plaque does not inherently possess negative attributes. It is a barrier that protects between the teeth and the acids that can harm them. Hence, certain individuals are capable of consuming substantial quantities of sugar without developing dental cavities. Provided that the pH level of the oral cavity remains within the alkaline threshold, the teeth are effectively shielded against the corrosive impact of the acids responsible for dental caries.

The mean urine pH is 6.0, however, it typically spans from 4.5 to 8.0. If urine pH levels drop below 5.0, it is regarded as acidic, whereas a urine pH above 8.0 is considered alkaline. The primary determinant of blood pH alteration is attributed to dietary intakes. An elevated urine pH level, indicating its alkalinity, may serve as an indicator of a potential medical condition such as a urinary tract infection, kidney infection, or the presence of kidney stones. Persistent emesis or diarrhea can result in an elevation of pH in urine, as these processes facilitate the expulsion of excessive gastric acid from the body, subsequently increasing the basicity of bodily fluids. A decrease in urine pH, indicative of an acidic urine environment, could be indicative of conditions such as diarrhea, malnutrition, or diabetic ketoacidosis, a potentially life-threatening complication associated with diabetes. The analysis of urine pH is commonly employed as a diagnostic tool to aid physicians in identifying potential underlying health conditions.

Litmus paper, a specially processed substrate, is immersed into the urine sample, subsequently leading to a perceptible change in the paper's hue. The hue is assessed in relation to a predetermined color palette, which subsequently determines the acidity or alkalinity of the urine. The individual should abstain from consuming food or beverages, or engaging in oral hygiene practices such as toothbrushing, for a minimum duration of thirty minutes prior to the examination in order to allow the saliva to be accurately analyzed. A small amount of saliva is expelled into a spoon or another container, followed by the examination of the saliva using a litmus paper test strip. Similar to the urine, the color of the test strip is altered and subsequently matched against a predefined chart to determine the acidity or basicity of the saliva. The acidity level of the blood is assessed in a comparable manner during the process of a blood test.

Understanding the pH level of the body is crucial for maintaining optimal health and ensuring the body remains balanced. Maintaining an optimal body pH level is crucial for preserving optimal bone health. Determining the state of the bones is inherently challenging as a result of the absence of any viable methods for conducting bone testing. The sole definitive means of discerning the possibility of bone weakness lies in the observation of fractured teeth or receding gum tissues; however, these indicators themselves do not suffice as the most reliable gauges of bone weakness.

This highlights the significant importance of regularly employing a pH test to assess the pH level of the body as a crucial measure in maintaining optimal bone health. Conducting periodic assessments of the body's pH level will provide valuable insight into the progression towards metabolic acidosis, or the extent to which the body is maintaining the essential equilibrium of mild alkalinity required for optimal bone health. The examination is straightforward and conveniently applicable within the comfort of one's own residence. It is readily achievable to obtain a trustworthy estimation of the pH level of the body's tissue by evaluating the pH level of the saliva or urine upon awakening in the morning.

MEASURE YOUR SALIVA

It is recommended that you perform the saliva test every morning upon waking up, prior to consuming anything or engaging in oral hygiene activities such as brushing your teeth. Commence by expelling all of the saliva present in your oral cavity. Please procure fresh saliva and consume it.

Perform this action twice more as you assemble your plastic or paper strip. When you generate saliva for the third time, expel it onto the strip and promptly observe the hue of the strip and its corresponding value (intensity) on the color chart. Aligning these colors will facilitate the determination of the pH value.

According to medical professionals, the ideal salivary pH level upon waking up should fall within the range of 6.2 to 6.8. Subsequently, this value tends to rise towards alkaline levels of 7.2 to 7.4 during the daytime.

One potential drawback of this method is that the pH of saliva may be influenced by the previous meal consumed before the test. What is the primary rationale behind the imperative to conduct the test as a matter of priority? It is important to acknowledge that while the paper strip is non-toxic, it is advisable to refrain from putting it in one's mouth.

Conducting a Urine Analysis is Now Required

The urine test is probably one of the best ways to to find out your pH level particularly if you require a somewhat accurate reading.

Once you awaken and before attending to your initial "short-call" of the day, it is advisable to wait until you have completed about half of the task. Subsequently, promptly immerse the pH test strip (whether made of paper or plastic) into the flow of urine and swiftly compare the resulting color on the strip to the corresponding color on the pH color chart.

In order to obtain precise outcomes, the velocity at which you observe can significantly impact the results. This phenomenon occurs due to the property of pHydron (the substance utilized in the production of the testing paper strips) that promotes evaporation. Any delay in conducting the test may lead to alterations in color, consequently leading to inaccurate outcomes. The ideal urine pH range should fall between 6.2 and 6.8.

In summation, it is imperative to recognize that relying solely on a single pH test is insufficient for determining the pH level of one's body. Various factors, including stress, dietary choices, and daily activities, have an impact on one's pH levels.

Hence, it is recommended to employ any of the aforementioned methods to assess your pH level. It is strongly recommended to perform multiple tests each day for a minimum of four consecutive days in order to ensure accuracy.

Chapter 4:

Sleep

You should possess an understanding of the paramount significance of obtaining sufficient and high-quality sleep in order to preserve and promote overall well-being. However, do you comprehend the reason behind that?

All phenomena on Earth are subject to cyclical and undulatory patterns. In a day, we possess a total of 24 hours, while we are graced with a span of 7 days in a week. We experience the phenomenon of alternating periods of darkness and light, brought about by the presence of the sun and moon, which are accompanied by the changing of seasons. The undulating pattern of oceanic waves corresponds to the ebb and flow of tides, which are influenced by the diurnal cycle.

Our physical beings also experience cyclical patterns. Our physical forms undergo physiological oscillations, particularly during the nocturnal period. In the period known as the late sleeping hours, which generally extends from after midnight until approximately 9 or

10 in the morning, the body undergoes a phase of detoxification. This phenomenon occurs when the human body actively expels accumulated acidity from its cells, tissues, and bloodstream, subsequently eliminating these toxic substances from the body.

The human body expels waste through the seven channels of elimination, namely the liver, lungs, lymphatic system, bloodstream, integumentary system, colon, and kidneys. For optimal well-being, the functionality of these elimination systems should be in good condition. The level of accumulation of toxins should be minimized.

There are several indications of the accumulation of toxicity, including:

Inadequate gastrointestinal function.

Insufficient availability of essential nutrients

Hepatic steatosis

Unexplained bouts of coughing

Difficulty in breathing

Unpleasant oral odor.

Systemic inflammation

Constant feelings of tiredness and fatigue throughout the entirety of the day.

Skin conditions such as acne, psoriasis, eczema, and inexplicable rashes may be observed.

Constipation and diarrhea

Symptoms of joint pain and rigidity

Renal calculi

Urine exhibiting a deep shade of yellow

Prominent, deep shadows beneath the eyes.

Envision a waterway replete with refuse and effluent. The contaminated water would exhibit a sluggish flow, leading to an obstruction of the river due to the accumulation of waste. This would result in the proliferation of bacteria, thus leading to a disruption of the ecological balance. This river would not possess the characteristics of robust health and vitality, teeming with abundant diverse forms of life.

The aforementioned statement applies to the internal circulation within your body as well. In order to maintain a robust circulation, it is imperative to ensure that the intake of toxins remains at a minimal level that can be effectively purified on a daily basis. By doing so, you can uphold a considerable degree of vitality.

Do you find yourself fatigued upon awakening from what should have been a rejuvenating night's sleep? Do you experience swollen eyes, halitosis, and tender joints? This is egregiously superfluous. You do not possess the attributes of a polluted river. You possess the inherent capacity to awaken with a sense of vigor and preparedness for the forthcoming day, exhibiting an appearance and demeanour that exudes vitality.

In order to attain this profound transformation, it will be necessary to evaluate the extent to which you are allocating time for relaxation and rejuvenation. Do you ensure that you allocate the necessary duration of 8 hours per night to enable your body to undergo the process of detoxification? Above all, what level of toxic exposure does your body endure throughout the course of the day? What are the filtration requirements of your systems during the nocturnal period, and to what extent does the accumulation of waste occur within your cells, tissues, and organs?

If you are experiencing bodily congestion, it is highly advisable to address and rectify the condition at present. Be ready to encounter initial discomforting symptoms. That which is ingested must inevitably be expelled. This is the functioning mechanism of the human body. Your physique demonstrates effective functioning, and by facilitating the natural restorative processes of the environment, all bodily systems will undergo detoxification.

Throughout the process of detoxification, you may encounter symptoms such as diarrhea, constipation, skin eruptions, halitosis, malodorous bowel movements, perspiration, coughing, and fatigue. This is a result of the internal cleansing procedure. Do not fret, this particular aspect of the process is of brief duration. One will be able to discern that the majority of the household cleaning has been completed when these indications cease to exist, and one's physical condition exhibits enhanced vitality. This can be attributed to an enhanced circulation of blood. You will gain the opportunity to witness the gradual disappearance of wrinkles and the enhanced vibrancy of color in your facial complexion. Your eyes will exhibit reduced swelling, enhanced clarity, and a vibrant appearance. Upon awakening, you will experience a revitalizing sensation accompanied by a pleasant sensation of freshness in your breath.

Having gained an understanding of the significance of sleep and the remarkable processes occurring within your body during this critical period, it is advisable that you demonstrate reverence for this essential aspect of your body's innate rhythms.

Strawberries

The immune system primarily derives benefits from the consumption of vitamin C contained in strawberries. In addition, they possess manganese, which facilitates the metabolic processes within our organism. Strawberries make an ideal inclusion in smoothies, and they lend themselves well to a diverse range of dessert preparations.

Apples

The consumption of one apple per day is believed to prevent the need for medical intervention. Although the adage may not be entirely accurate, apples remain highly beneficial for the human body from a health standpoint. They possess abundant quantities of vitamin C and flavonoids, a type of antioxidant that fortifies the immune system and aids in the prevention of cancer. In addition, they possess a significant quantity of dietary fiber that our bodies utilize for the purpose of detoxification.

Apples are a crucial component for maintaining optimal levels of cholesterol and blood pressure. An alternative option is to utilize apple cider vinegar, which offers additional benefits. Notably, it contains acetic acid, a nutrient that possesses antiviral and antibacterial properties, despite its nomenclature.

Watermelon

Watermelon supplies the body with essential electrolytes such as potassium, which play a crucial role in maintaining cardiovascular well-being. It plays a role in enhancing our body's hydration levels due to its abundant water content, as evident from its name. One may exercise ingenuity and concoct a watermelon smoothie, or alternatively, partake in this fruit as a refreshingly light snack.

Raisins

Should you experience a desire for sugar, consuming raisins may potentially assuage it. They are rich in antioxidants, and certain studies have demonstrated their potential to regulate blood pressure.

Garlic

There are individuals who assert that garlic possesses miraculous properties, and I can confidently affirm that their assertion is indeed accurate. It has the potential to enhance the functioning of your cardiovascular and immune systems, facilitate detoxification of your liver, and assist in the maintenance of healthy blood pressure levels.

Lemon

Similar to the orange, the lemon is renowned for its efficacy in combatting influenza and colds. These narratives are completely valid, as it is irrefutable that lemons effectively combat viruses within our biological system. Moreover, they possess the ability to promote wound healing, enhance hepatic function, and facilitate the detoxification process within the body.

Cayenne peppers

Cayenne peppers contain a substantial quantity of vitamin A, in addition to

refrain from consuming them, yet it is important to bear in mind the 80:20 proportion highlighted in the segment providing an overview of the alkaline diet.

Fruits and Veggies

Indeed, certain fruits and vegetables possess elevated levels of acidity, rendering them unsuitable for consumption within the confines of an alkaline diet. Regarding fruits, it is advisable to restrict the consumption of blueberries, currants, and cranberries. Similarly, glazed and canned fruits should be avoided altogether due to the addition of artificial preservatives and sweeteners in the majority of cases. Additionally, it should be taken into consideration that processed fruit juices possess a significant acidity level.

In regards to vegetables, it is important to be aware that lentils, olives, winter squash, and corn possess a significant level of acidity. While they do retain certain nutrients and fiber content, it is advisable to restrict their inclusion within your dietary regimen.

Dairy

Unfavorable developments arise for individuals who have an affinity for dairy products - their consumption should be limited within the context of the alkaline diet. One might question the reason behind this phenomenon, considering the ample calcium content, however, it must be acknowledged that the acidic nature of the substance outweighs the advantages it offers.

Regrettably, opting for low-fat variations of dairy products will not yield any significant changes. It is imperative to strictly curtail the consumption of certain food items, including various types of cheese, yogurt, milk, and butter, as part of a health-conscious dietary regimen. Similarly, the aforementioned applies to eggs, particularly their yolks, which exhibit elevated levels of acidity as well.

Grains

The issue concerning grains pertains to the fact that during the process of baking and processing, the valuable compounds contained within them are depleted, resulting in the production of excessively acidic products. Furthermore, it should be noted that these products have a limited quantity of essential nutrients and dietary fiber, which in itself is a compelling reason to avoid consuming them.

Grains that necessitate restriction consist of white bread, pasta, and doughnuts. Assortment of bagels, assorted pastries, biscuits, crackers, and refined white rice.

Meat

Indeed, meat can serve as a significant provider of proteins. However, it is crucial to note that upon protein metabolism, it is classified as acidic. The cause of this can be attributed to purines, the chemical constituents that give rise to uric acid. This not only has an acidifying impact on our internal pH levels, but it can also disseminate to joints and tissues, leading to complications such as renal calculi and gout.

That does not imply that you ought to completely refrain from consuming meat. Please bear in mind the principle of an 80:20 ratio favoring highly alkaline foods, while also ensuring that your meat selection consistently consists of free-range and organic options, as they tend to possess enhanced nutrient content.

Nuts and Oils

When seeking a protein source to incorporate into our diet, nuts present a superior alternative to meat and other animal-derived products. The explanation can be attributed to the lower acidity levels experienced by plants when metabolized, which serves as the underlying cause. Nevertheless, with the exception of hazelnuts, the majority of them still exhibit an acidifying impact, thus necessitating their consumption in moderation.

Regarding oils, sunflower seed and canola oil, much like other vegetable oils, possess a moderately elevated acidity level. Furthermore, it is not implied that complete avoidance of these substances is necessary; rather, it is advisable to exercise restraint in their consumption.

Refined Sugar

We have now arrived at an element that is strongly discouraged in the alkaline diet (as well as in any other sound nutritional regimen). Refined sugar exhibits high acidity levels, making it a prominent factor contributing to the elevated internal pH levels observed in individuals. The human body expends significant effort in counteracting the acidifying consequences brought about by processed sugar, rendering it unnecessary to subject the body to such labor.

Exclusively abstain from consuming muffins, sodas, candy, pastries, and other comestibles commonly perceived as indulgent.

Coffee

The inclusion of this item on the list is likely to be met with disappointment among coffee enthusiasts. All varieties of coffee exhibit excessive acidity;

however, if one desires to indulge in an infrequent cup or two, it is imperative to opt for a type such as Swiss water decaffeinated coffee, which possesses a reduced overall acidity level.

Alcohol

Notwithstanding its caloric content, alcohol is strictly proscribed in the alkaline diet due to its excessively acidic nature. It has the potential to deplete vital minerals, such as magnesium, from your body, and may induce gastric discomfort in individuals who exhibit sensitivity to highly acidic dietary items.

Here are additional recommendations for restricting and abstaining from certain foods within the context of adhering to an alkaline diet:

Please ensure to avoid the consumption of food preservatives as well as artificial sweeteners and coloring. Consuming any food containing these ingredients is strongly discouraged due to its highly detrimental health effects.

Refrain from indiscriminate use of antibiotics or pharmaceuticals, unless explicitly prescribed by medical professionals.

Refrain from ingesting your food hastily. Rather, make an effort to chew the food thoroughly, as this will further aid in reducing the acidity levels in the body.

Eating Out Guide

I have yet to encounter an individual who does not derive occasional pleasure from dining outside of their home. The cause potentially resides within the social factor, as dining out typically entails gathering with friends and enjoying a pleasant experience. When commencing the implementation of an alkaline diet, one may encounter certain obstacles in maintaining adherence while dining outside of the home. That should not imply or suggest that you should abstain from socializing with your acquaintances. If you carefully review the guidelines we have meticulously assembled for your convenience, you will effortlessly navigate dining at a restaurant while maintaining an optimal equilibrium of your internal pH levels.

Initially, it is imperative that you engage in adequate research prior to embarking on your endeavors. One may demonstrate foresight and conduct preliminary investigations into the dining establishments within their vicinity that are reputed for their emphasis on maintaining good health. As an alternative, consider perusing the menus available on their websites and preselecting the main course that aligns with your alkaline dietary preferences.

One additional point to consider is that it would be advisable not to experience hunger prior to visiting the restaurant. By doing so, you will be more likely to succumb to the temptation of sampling the excessively acidic cuisine available. An effective solution to this issue would be to consume a light food item prior to your departure.

Upon your arrival at the restaurant, kindly proceed to place an order for a salad comprising a selection of fresh and crisp leafy greens. This will serve two purposes - it will elevate your alkalinity levels and result in earlier satiety. There is no requisite to feel compelled to also partake in the main course. You have the option to select two appetizers instead. To illustrate this point, upon completion of the salad course, it is permissible to request a vegetable soup as an alternative option.

If you decide to place an order for an entrée, salmon would be suitably fitting. Please ensure that you inquire about the freshness of the fish and its origin, specifically if it is wild-caught or farm-raised (the former being the preferable choice). It is advisable to abstain from consuming fried food, as well as grains, such as the bread that may be served by the waiter. Please take note that dining establishments frequently offer the option to select accompanying dishes, affording you the opportunity to opt for vegetables or leafy greens.

Regarding the dessert, it might be prudent to entirely forgo it. This phenomenon can be attributed to the prevalence of refined sugar and high caloric content found in restaurant desserts.

When considering beverage options, it is advisable to opt for herbal tea and water as more preferable alternatives to sugary drinks, which should be abstained from. A similar principle applies to coffee, however, if consumption is necessary, it is advisable to restrict oneself to a single serving.

Below are additional suggestions that you may find helpful while dining at restaurants:

Please feel free to engage in communication with the waiter. Ultimately, it would behoove him to acknowledge that he stands to receive a considerable gratuity by exerting effort to address any inquiries and fulfill any requests made by you. If he has been nothing but amicable towards you, ensure that you express gratitude by offering a suitable gratuity.

You may approach one of your acquaintances to partake in a communal meal. That is an effective method for regulating portion size and consuming a reduced quantity of food.

Kindly request the waiter to serve the condiments separately. By doing so, you can exercise greater control over the amount of dressing utilized in your salad while ensuring the avoidance of any detrimental ingredients, such as mayonnaise.

Please allocate sufficient time for masticating your food, similar to how you would savor your meals at home, in order to fully enjoy the experience and consume your meal gradually.

It is advisable to refrain from consuming excessive amounts of salt, as it is often readily available on restaurant tables for additional seasoning purposes. Nevertheless, these options typically do not provide a healthy amount of salt, therefore it would be advisable to refrain from consuming them.

127

The Rise of Acidity

Western diets exhibit a significant prevalence of high acidity levels. There is speculation suggesting that this could potentially be one of the contributing factors to the high prevalence of cancer in the current era. Irrespective of the veracity of this statement, it is unequivocally established that an excessively acidic constitution is detrimental to one's overall well-being.

As we explore the alkaline diet, it is imperative to initially discern the categorization of foods to abstain from based on their elevated acidic composition.

Alcohol

Whilst red wine does offer certain health benefits, it is imperative to exercise moderation when consuming any form of alcohol due to its elevated acid content. Certain wines exhibit pH levels close to 3.5. In the event that alcohol consumption is a recurrent component of one's dietary habits, it has the potential to induce an acidifying effect on the body.

Artificial Sweeteners

Most health experts concur that substances such as Aspartame and Sucralose are commonly regarded as misleading byproducts. In addition to other concerns and potential neurological implications stemming from aspartame, it is noteworthy that these substances also possess acidity. Watch out!

Animal Meat

Embarking on an alkaline diet further entails the elimination of meat from one's dietary choices. The vast majority of animal proteins exhibit an acidic nature. The acidity is heightened when animal protein is deep-fried using oils that are even more acidic or combined with white pasta dishes.

Bananas

Bananas can be utilized as a delicious ingredient to add substance in various recipes, however, it is advisable to refrain from consuming them as standalone snacks due to their elevated acid content and comparatively lower nutrient profile in comparison to alternative fruits.

Berries

Certain types of berries display a higher level of acidity, exemplified by raspberries and blueberries. Additional fruits that can be classified as acidic include currants, plums, and prunes.

Black Tea

Similar to coffee, its acidity level is remarkably high. If you have a preference for black teas, it is important to ensure a sufficient intake of alkalizing food to maintain balance.

Certain Nuts

Certain nuts can be seamlessly integrated into alkaline-based recipes without imparting any detrimental effects. Nevertheless, indulging in an excessive quantity of nuts, particularly those high in sodium content, in isolation can result in a reduction in the pH level of your body. This encompasses cashews, peanuts, and almonds.

Chocolate

A difficult one to relinquish. Chocolate possesses a notable acidic profile in all its variations. The inexpensive processed milk chocolates, perhaps even more so than raw and unprocessed dark chocolates and cacao. The optimal approach in this particular scenario would be to maintain the overall balance of your diet at an increased level of alkalinity, thereby allowing you to continue indulging in chocolate or incorporating it into your culinary preparations.

Coffee

I am aware that the media frequently oscillates between portraying coffee as beneficial and as detrimental to one's health. On one occasion, it exhibits curative properties against cancer, while on another occasion, it is attributed to the onset of heart disease. It is the case that coffee is not lethal, however it possesses a significantly high acidic content. Having a single cup might not have significant consequences, but if incorporated into your everyday dietary routine, it becomes an issue.

Cooking Oils

Typical culinary oils, such as corn and sunflower varieties that are less expensive, connote a relatively acidic composition.

Corn

This vegetable can be described as lacking in substantive nutritional value, as it contains primarily starch and sugar with minimal additional nutritional components. Due to its acidic nature, it would be prudent to restrict or eliminate the consumption of corn from your dietary intake.

Most Dairy

The majority of milk and cheese products exhibit a pH level that varies from mildly acidic to neutral (such as cream and yogurt) and can extend to highly acidic range. To illustrate, parmesan cheese exhibits significantly higher acidity compared to other types of cheese, resulting in an elevated renal load of acidity. Furthermore, it should be noted that pasteurized cheeses from the United States generally exhibit pH levels of approximately 5, a markedly higher acidity when compared to other types of cheeses.

Processed Sugary Crap

Corn syrups, molasses, and artificially processed honey are all contributors to the acidification of the body. It is imperative that you commence immediately with the elimination of them.

Soft Drinks

There are numerous justifications for abstaining from consuming soft drinks (sodas). Another factor can be attributed to their high acidity. If you are embarking on an alkaline diet, it is advised to entirely eliminate soft drinks, carbonated syrup drinks, and similar beverages from your dietary intake. The pH level of Coca Cola is remarkably low at 2. This substance exhibits a distinctly high level of acidity.

Sodium

In addition to elevating blood pressure, highly salted foods also contribute to an increase in acidity levels. Make an effort to minimize the use of sodium in your culinary preparations, and avoid indulging in salty snacks such as chips or nuts. Similarly, exercise caution when consuming sauces and dressings that have a high salt content. As an illustration, soy sauce may serve as an appropriate example.

Sweets and Desserts

Consuming candy bars, caramel, and other types of junk food can be detrimental to one's well-being. There exist numerous compelling reasons, ranging from the excessive presence of saturated fat to the utilization of high fructose corn syrup, which warrant the avoidance of such items. Furthermore, it is worth noting that they possess high acidity levels.

White Bread and the majority of Grain Products

White bread has a pH level of 5, denoting substantial acidity. This encompasses white pastas and other types of simple carbohydrates as well. There exist numerous additional rationales for steering clear of these, comprising weight acquisition, as well as the manner in which they abruptly elevate your blood sugar, leading to subsequent energy crashes and diminished levels of vitality. Consecutive episodes of sugar crashes also lead to an increase in hunger, resulting in a distressing situation for individuals pursuing a controlled dietary regimen.

Aside from white bread, the majority of grains possess an acidic nature. Hence, a balanced alkaline diet restricts the consumption of grains. Nevertheless, it is not necessary to entirely eliminate them. Certain varieties of cereal grains, particularly those abundant with nutritious nuts and seeds, are recommended for consumption and should continue to be incorporated into one's diet.

It is worth noting that there exists a comprehensive perspective advocating for the complete elimination of ALL GRAINS from our dietary intake. I have chosen not to incorporate this philosophy into this cookbook, as the alkaline diet, which is primarily vegan, already encompasses a substantial portion of its principles. Additionally, excluding grains from the recipes would excessively restrict our culinary choices and potentially compromise the overall dining experience. Nevertheless, it is possible to achieve nutritional adequacy by adhering to a disciplined approach (please refer to my publications on the RAW FOOD DIET).

The Mechanisms of the Alkaline Diet

The alkaline diet can be viewed as the antithesis of the prevailing dietary trend characterized by high fat, high protein, and low carbohydrate intake. If you are unfamiliar with the concept of an alkaline diet, you are not alone; however, it may prove advantageous for you.

If one experiences discomfort after consuming a low carbohydrate, high protein diet, it is advisable to contemplate adopting the alkaline diet. You should additionally take into consideration whether you exhibit symptoms indicative of heightened acidity. The aforementioned indications encompass persistent fatigue, diminished vitality, nasal congestion, recurrent infections or colds, feelings of nervousness, anxiety, or stress, parched hair and/or skin, brittle nails, muscular discomfort, leg spasms, outbreaks of hives, and inflammation of the stomach lining, also known as gastritis.

Prior to initiation, it is advisable to assess the pH level of your saliva to determine its current state. If the pH level is significantly low, such as a 4, then this indicates an acidic outcome. If the pH level is elevated, such as reaching a value of 8, then it can be characterized as being alkaline. After obtaining the knowledge of your pH level as well as the distinction between alkaline and acidic foods, you can commence the process of equilibrium and ensure the continuous alkaline pH state of your body.

There are multiple freely accessible charts accessible on the internet that can offer comprehensive information. Let us examine a selection of alkaline fruits, including bananas, apples, coconut, nectarines, pineapple, and tomatoes, to name but a few. Alfalfa, celery, cabbage, carrots, garlic, lettuce, and mushrooms can be considered as some examples of alkaline vegetables. In addition, there are alkaline dairy products, cereals, and nuts.

How does it work? The majority of foods can be classified as either alkaline or acidic based on the residual impact they have on the body and their metabolic processes. It would be advantageous to pursue a state of bodily equilibrium with a subtle alkaline nature. It is advisable not to make assumptions about the acidity or alkalinity of one's diet solely based on the food consumed. There are numerous factors that can influence the pH levels of the human body. A case in point is the phenomenon where the acidity of an orange transforms into alkalinity upon consumption.

Following an alkaline diet that maintains a slightly alkaline state in the body can contribute to enhancing one's general well-being. It has been speculated that it may possess the ability to inhibit the development of cancer cells, and an alkaline diet has demonstrated the potential to enhance the potency and efficacy of certain chemotherapy drugs. It has the potential to assist in the restoration of your well-being and ensure an absence of ailments. It has the ability to replenish energy and vitality, and alleviate nasal congestion, headache, as well as joint and muscular discomfort.

Despite the limited availability of direct research on the alkaline diet, ample evidence exists to establish a correlation between individuals who frequently fall ill and their tendency to have acidic blood, indicating an imbalance. Rarely does blood exhibit excessive alkalinity, thus there is no cause for concern regarding the consumption of an abundance of alkaline foods.

What are the Effects of Acidity on the Human Body? To address this inquiry, consider envisioning the human body as a recipient of diverse food substances. The consumption of various foods, irrespective of their acidic or alkaline properties, induces a chemical response that regulates the overall pH level within the body. Having an acidic nature indicates that the pH level of our body is below the optimal range. The pH range that is considered optimal is approximately 7.35-7.45, indicating a slight alkaline state. This environment optimally supports cellular function and promotes robust immune response against pathogenic ailments. Currently, the pH of our blood maintains a range between 7.35 and 7.45 within our body, and it is exceedingly rare for it to decrease below 7.35. However, in the event that the pH level does drop below 7.35, it leads to the occurrence of acidosis. Essentially, in order to maintain a constant alkalinity level (pH ranging from 7.35 to 7.45) and prevent the onset of acidosis, the body must extract minerals from our bones as minerals possess alkaline properties.

This is the reason why individuals may experience osteoporosis, degenerative diseases, and tumors, as the body's response to maintain alkalinity in the blood becomes disrupted. Indicators of heightened acidity levels include diminished energy levels and persistent fatigue, an excessive generation of mucus, nasal blockage, persistent viral ailments and infections, apprehension, stress, irritability, brittle nails, weakened hair, parched skin, ovarian cysts, benign breast cysts, polycystic ovaries, migraines, arthritis, neuritis, muscle discomfort, hives, cramps, spasms, dyspepsia, and gastritis. An increasing body of research indicates that individuals with lower, or acidic, pH levels are correlated with an elevated likelihood of developing conditions such as type 2 diabetes, heart disease, and obesity. The alkaline diets present remedies to address these issues through their detoxifying properties. The detoxification properties possess the capacity to purify the bloodstream and rejuvenate cellular structures within the organism. Yeast, bacteria, fungus, and viruses require acidic environments in order to flourish and proliferate. Nonetheless, this is not the situation in

Alkaline-based environments. The Alkaline Diet provides a substantial reduction in the likelihood of encountering these issues. The consumption of food in Alkaline Diets is noteworthy for its ability to cleanse the kidneys and prevent the occurrence of assorted kidney-related ailments. Incorporating food into one's daily dietary intake presents a significant reservoir of calcium, thereby providing a viable alternative to numerous calcium supplements. Moreover, it incorporates a substantial quantity of sodium, which facilitates the process of digestion. These examples only scratch the surface of the various functions food fulfills within the framework of Alkaline Diets.

A research study carried out at the University of California, involving a sample size of 9,000 women, revealed that individuals with chronic acidosis are considerably more susceptible to experiencing bone loss when compared to individuals with normal pH levels. The researchers involved in this experiment posit that a substantial portion of the hip fractures prevalent among women in their middle years can be attributed to elevated acidity levels. This is attributed to a diet characterized by inadequate vegetable consumption and excessive intake of animal-based products. The rationale for this phenomenon lies in the fact that the human body utilizes calcium from our skeletal system to maintain equilibrium in pH levels.

Ensuring equilibrium in your pH level encompasses more than simply selecting alkaline foods for consumption. The majority of individuals believed that a mere consumption of alkaline foods would prove adequate, resulting in the restoration of their pH level to its optimal state.

However, this assertion couldn't be farther from reality. To effectively initiate your alkaline diet, it is imperative to possess precise knowledge regarding the optimal method of assimilating all essential nutrients, minerals, and vitamins.

What is PH level

The abbreviation PH stands for "potential of hydrogen" and is employed to quantify the acidity levels of cells and various other substances. The acidity scale spans from 0 to 14, with the ideal pH value for the body typically falling within the center of this range. A majority of over 90% of the American population exhibits an acidic pH level as a consequence of dietary choices, insufficient hydration, elevated stress levels, and various other contributing factors. The pH scale quantifies the acidity level of an aqueous solution. Considering that the human body predominantly comprises water, the pH level can be employed to characterize the acidity levels present in bodily fluids. The pH value of water is measured at 7.0. When the pH falls below 7, it indicates an acidic nature, whereas when the pH exceeds 7, it signifies basic or alkaline properties. Our physiological systems sustain a blood pH level of approximately 7.4. The renal system ensures the meticulous regulation of this pH equilibrium through the perpetual filtration of acids and bases in the circulatory system. The kidneys eliminate an appropriate quantity of acid or base in the urine to maintain the body's pH equilibrium. Other particular bodily fluids exhibit high acidity (such as gastric acid) or alkalinity (enzymatic fluids present in the pancreas). These fluids are vigilantly confined, ensuring their separation from the bloodstream and bodily tissues to prevent any potential harm that may arise from their inadvertent release. The gastrointestinal system—While the oral cavity serves as the primary gateway for ingested substances, the digestive system often begins preparing itself even prior to the initial ingestion. How is food digested. The process of digestion encompasses the amalgamation of food, its propulsion through the digestive tract, and the enzymatic degradation of complex food constituents into simpler molecular components. The process of digestion commences within the oral cavity as we engage in mastication and subsequently swallow, ultimately reaching its culmination within the small intestine. The gastrointestinal system comprises the physiological components that collaborate harmoniously to convert food and beverages into the essential elemental constituents and energy required by the body. Most gastrointestinal disorders, such as dyspepsia, emesis, distension, gastroesophageal reflux, manifest as symptoms resulting from an abundance of acidic content in the gastric region and an insufficiency of alkaline minerals in the intestinal tract. In the event that the enzyme-dense foods lack the presence of alkaline minerals, the pancreas will experience fatigue. Consequently, when the pancreas reaches a state of exhaustion, it consequently forfeits its capacity to interpret and direct the body's response to ingested food. This phenomenon will result in a progressive deterioration through a descent into disorder, causing organs to undergo disorientation and inflammation. The circulatory system can be attributed to heart disease primarily caused by elevated levels of acidity. It is widely acknowledged that numerous fats play a crucial and indispensable role in maintaining cardiovascular well-being. Healthy fats, in fact, possess the capability to alleviate the inflammation that serves as the root cause of arteriosclerosis. When the arteries undergo a condition of plaque-induced thickening, it is not attributed to the presence of beneficial fats but rather arises from the inflammatory responses triggered by the internal acidic milieu. The human body reacts to the acidic environment by forming fatty deposits along the blood vessels to avoid any potentially fatal ruptures, a process that halts the imminent threat of death. However, this places burden on the heart due to the resulting constriction in the blood flow pathway. When the heart reaches a state of complete tiredness, it is referred to as a myocardial infarction. Your circulatory system constitutes a intricate arrangement of various organs and vessels that facilitate the efficient transportation of nutrients, blood, hormones, and oxygen to and from cellular entities. In the absence of your circulatory system, your body's ability to maintain a healthy internal environment and defend against diseases is compromised. Typically, the physiological organs contribute to the preservation of appropriate pH and temperature levels within your body with the aim of promoting wellness.

The immune system is a sophisticated network of cellular components that collaborate to safeguard the body from intrusive or foreign cells, encompassing those that may be atypical and potentially give rise to malignancies. The majority of intruders from foreign sources are microorganisms known as pathogens, which encompass infection-causing entities like harmful bacteria. Within your body, there exists a sophisticated mechanism specifically tailored to safeguard you from countless bacteria, microbes, viruses, toxins, and parasites. Although these protective systems operate diligently to ensure our well-being, many of us possess limited understanding of the functions and workings of the immune system. Having a comprehensive understanding of scientific concepts is not essential, but possessing a rudimentary grasp of the subject matter can aid in comprehending variations, ailments such as the flu and common cold, and associated symptoms. Considering the extensive impact of the immune system on various bodily functions, it is unsurprising that immune system functionality or malfunction is a pervasive concern in nearly all diseases. The immune system is also involved in the development and progression of cancer. As the immune system loses its ability to recognize and eliminate tumor cells, the conditions become favorable for the development of cancers and tumors. Despite extensive knowledge gained by scientists regarding the immune system, their ongoing focus remains on investigating the mechanisms through which the body successfully initiates defense mechanisms aimed at eliminating invading microorganisms, infected cells, and tumors, while simultaneously avoiding damage to healthy tissues. Recent advancements in technology have now empowered scientists to swiftly ascertain the specific stimuli inciting an immunological response by means of identifying individual immune cells. Advancements in microscopy techniques are facilitating the unprecedented examination of B cells, T cells, and other cellular entities in their dynamic interactions within lymph nodes and various anatomical tissues.

The immune system safeguards our well-being by recognizing specific molecules present on the surface of our cells, known as Human Leukocyte Antigens (HLA molecules), which serve as indicators to affirm their affiliation with the body. These molecules exhibit the highest degree of variability among human proteins, thereby resulting in individuals possessing a unique combination that distinguishes their

"HLA type" from others. When medical professionals engage in discussions regarding transplant compatibility, they are essentially referring to the correlation between HLA types of the donor and recipient, as any disparity in HLA molecules may induce rejection of the transplant.

Respiratory system - Inhalation is the physiological mechanism through which atmospheric oxygen is conveyed into the pulmonary system, subsequently facilitating the transportation of oxygen throughout the organism. Our pulmonary system extracts oxygen from the atmosphere and subsequently transports it via the circulatory system to the various tissues and organs responsible for facilitating locomotion, speech, and motion. Our respiratory system additionally extracts carbon dioxide from our bloodstream and expels it into the atmosphere during exhalation. When the tissues and organs undergo acid overload, the transportation of oxygen is significantly impaired. This state of asphyxiation results in impaired cellular respiration. In order for all cells within our organism to operate in optimal conditions, it is imperative for them to receive a fresh supply of oxygen and expel accumulated carbon dioxide, which has an acidic nature. Excessive acidity levels trigger the accumulation of mucous, infections, and viruses within our respiratory system, ultimately giving rise to various respiratory ailments such as common colds, bronchitis, and asthma.

Arthritis falls under the classification of rheumatic diseases. These are distinct medical conditions, each characterized by varying symptoms, treatment methods, potential complications, and long-term outlook. They share a common characteristic of impacting the joints, muscles, ligaments, cartilage, and tendons, along with the potential to impact internal bodily regions. Rheumatoid and Osteoarthritis are the two primary manifestations of arthritis. Both forms are associated with an imbalance in pH levels and the buildup of acidic deposits in the joints and wrists. The detrimental impact on cartilage is caused by the accumulation of this acid. When the cellular activity responsible for the production of synovial and bursa fluids is characterized by acidity, it gives rise to a state of dryness within the joints which subsequently leads to irritation and swelling. These conditions can be reversed by adhering to a suitable alkaline diet. Specifically, we refer to the Integumentary system, more commonly recognized as the skin. When the body's pH is imbalanced, an accumulation of acidic substances leads to inflammation, undermining the skin's ability to serve as an innate defense mechanism against infections. The Integumentary System comprises the body's largest organ, namely, the skin. This remarkable anatomical system serves the purpose of safeguarding the internal structures of the body against harm, averting desiccation, storing lipid reserves, while concurrently generating essential vitamins and hormones. Additionally, it aids in the maintenance of homeostasis within the body through its role in regulating both body temperature and water balance. The integumentary system serves as the initial barrier to protect the body from bacterial, viral, and other pathogenic invasions. Additionally, it assists in offering safeguard against detrimental ultraviolet radiation. The skin serves as a sensory organ by possessing receptors that can perceive variations in temperature.

The nervous system can be described as a sophisticated network of nerves and specialized cells called neurons, which facilitate the transmission of signals across various regions of the body. It serves as the fundamental network for the transmission of electrical signals within the human body. The excessive acid levels can adversely impact the vitality of the nervous system by depriving it of essential energy resources. This phenomenon can also be referred to as "devitalizing" or "enervation." It induces physical, psychological, and emotional debilitation.

157

The excretory system functions as a passive biological mechanism that facilitates the elimination of surplus and superfluous substances from the bodily fluids of an organism. It closely collaborates with both the circulatory and endocrine systems. The connection pertaining to the circulatory system is readily apparent. The blood that is circulated throughout the body traverses one of the two kidneys. The kidneys are responsible for extracting urea, uric acid, and water from the bloodstream, while a majority of the water is subsequently reintroduced to the system. This bodily function entails the filtration and purification of fluids within our blood. In the event that an excessive concentration of acids overwhelms the body, compensatory mechanisms are activated, one of which involves the extraction of alkaline minerals from the skeletal system and their subsequent release into the bloodstream. In the event of frequent occurrences, the minerals accumulate within the kidneys, manifesting as renal calculi that cause a considerable amount of discomfort.

The muscular system consists of numerous specialized cells. They possess anatomical compositions that have been specifically adapted to fulfill their respective purposes. An illustrative instance would be when muscle cells facilitate the convergence of bodily components. They consist of protein fibers that have the ability to contract in response to energy availability, causing the cells to shorten. There exist three distinct types of muscle, with skeletal muscles alone being under voluntary control, signifying conscious regulation. Smooth and cardiac muscles exhibit involuntary contractions. Smooth and cardiac muscles demonstrate automatic contractions. Smooth and cardiac muscles engage in spontaneous contractions. Smooth and cardiac muscles demonstrate unplanned contractions.

Each category of muscles within the muscular system serves a distinct function. You possess the capability to ambulate due to the functioning of your skeletal muscles. The process of digestion is made possible due to the presence of smooth muscles within your body. Your cardiac muscle is responsible for the beating of your heart. The various types of muscles also collaborate to facilitate the execution of these functions. As an illustration, during the act of running (involving skeletal muscles), the cardiac muscle facilitates increased pumping action of the heart, leading to heightened respiration (involving smooth muscles). There exists a plethora of diseases and disorders that are correlated with an acidic state, including but not limited to cataracts, osteoporosis, gout, cancer, migraines, constipation, morning sickness, stroke, allergies, diabetes, and obesity. With this consciousness regarding the impact of acidity on our well-being, individuals can exercise the ability to make knowledgeable and prudent choices regarding the dietary components that contribute to maintaining a state of optimal health for our bodies.

Additional Health Advantages of an Alkaline Diet

Consuming alkaline foods enhances both the immune system and energy levels, as they possess abundant antioxidants and fiber. By maintaining an understanding of the difference between acid and alkaline foods, you will be able to make informed decisions. Some advantages of consuming alkaline food are:

• Muscle mass and bone density: Your body requires minerals to ensure the maintenance of robust and healthy skeletal structures. Based on research findings, the consumption of alkalized vegetables and fruits has been shown to provide a protective effect against muscle wasting and the deterioration of bone strength. The alkaline diet helps maintain appropriate levels of essential minerals, including phosphate, magnesium, and calcium, which contribute to the development of muscle

161

mass and bone strength. The diet also has a beneficial impact on the absorption of vitamin D and the production of growth hormones, thereby providing further protection to the bones and reducing the likelihood of developing chronic complications.

• In order to enhance the effects of anti-aging, decrease inflammation, and stimulate the production of growth hormone in the body, it is advisable to limit the consumption of acidic foods when following alkaline diets, as this can help prevent strokes and high blood pressure. You will experience improved cardiovascular well-being that effectively safeguards against prevalent medical conditions such as hypertension, memory loss, cerebrovascular incidents, nephrolithiasis, and elevated levels of cholesterol, which affect a significant proportion of the global population.

• In the context of inflammation and chronic pain, the alkaline diet has demonstrated efficacy in reducing levels of persistent pain. Multiple research studies have demonstrated notable diminishment of pain among individuals suffering from chronic back pain after undergoing trials involving the administration of alkaline supplements.

• Enhanced magnesium levels and improved vitamin consumption: In order for optimal bodily functioning to be achieved, an adequate intake of magnesium is necessary. The alkaline diet enhances the absorption of magnesium. Magnesium deficiency is prevalent among individuals who suffer from ailments such as muscular discomfort, cardiac issues, anxiety, sleep disturbances, and headaches. Additionally, it is necessary to supplement with magnesium in order to enhance your immune system by increasing your intake of vitamin D.

• Cancer prevention: The alkaline diet has garnered significant attention due to its potential to protect against the development of cancer. According to research findings, it has been observed that cancerous cells exhibit a higher rate of mortality in an organism with a more alkaline internal environment. It has additionally been determined that an alkaline phrase enhances the efficiency of chemotherapy medicaments. In addition, alkalinity reduces inflammation, enhances our immune system, and mitigates the occurrence and potential hazards associated with cancer.

• Optimal weight: The alkaline diet exerts influence on the accumulation of weight and the issue of obesity. The diet restricts the consumption of acidic foods and promotes the ingress of alkaline foods that are essential for our daily nourishment. By refraining from consuming foods that lead to acid formation in the body, one can effectively reduce levels of leptin and enhance the body's capacity to metabolize fat. In addition, it should be noted that alkaline foods such as spinach, celery, and butternut squash exhibit exceptional nutritional density, possess potent anti-inflammatory properties, and boast low-caloric content.

Now, let us proceed to discuss the methods of incorporating these plants into some delectable alkaline recipes.